HABITS TO AVOID

Oneself Free from negative habits

TABLE OF CONTENTS

INTRODUCTION

It's not a good idea to degrade yourself because you have fallen victim to undesirable habits. These habits affect everyone in their life. Yet in real life, the winner is the one who can admit their error and break harmful behaviors.

You become aware of how simple it is to succumb to a long list of unhealthy behaviors when you examine your lifestyle. Becoming oneself free from negative habits and breaking them is the difficult part.

At first glance, habits like biting your nails or fidgeting with your hair while you're awake may seem harmless, but over time, they can be challenging to quit. Coupled with this, unhealthy behaviors like smoking and drinking are terrible for your health.

At first glance, habits like biting your nails or fidgeting with your hair while you're awake may seem harmless, but over time, they can be challenging to quit. Coupled with this, unhealthy behaviors like smoking and drinking are terrible for your health.

Cancer and lung illness can result from these two behaviors. The best course of action in this circumstance is to kick these negative habits by leading a normal life. You should immediately stop some of the unhealthy behaviors we've identified in this post.

At first glance, habits like biting your nails or fidgeting with your hair while you're awake may seem harmless, but over time, they can be challenging to quit. In addition to this, several unhealthy habits are terrible for, as with drinking and smoking, your health.

Bad Habits to Break Immediately
As I previously stated, the way of life we choose leads to the development of negative habits. The most crucial thing is to identify which negative habits are actually harmful to your life before taking the required efforts to break them. Let's examine a few of these behaviors below:

1. Being tardy

On a regular basis, some people are late. This inclination might negatively impact your life. The first is that it might force you to put things off.

They never take you at your word and always anticipate you to be late. They might conclude from this that you are unreliable. Also, being late can be harmful to you because you have developed the poor habit of never being on time, which can make it challenging for you to get somewhere in time.

The best way to break this bad habit is to realize the importance of time.

2. Being overly critical of yourself

There will be occasions when you simply can't finish your assignment by the deadline. It can be due to a work emergency, a family emergency, or another emergency. If that's the case, try not to dwell on it. That's just the way things are at times.

What can you do, then? Grab your attention back. Continue your job where you left off and pick up where you left off. Complaining will not solve your problems.

3. Spending time with individuals who don't value you

The human mind is wired to yearn for those who value you. Your life may go worse if you spend time with people who don't value you. This is such a negative habit that it might cause you to perform below your ability and underestimate yourself.

Making friends with individuals who value you for who you are is the best way to break this terrible behavior. Watch out for those who give you honest praise and strive to make you a better person. To stop this unhealthy habit of contaminating your brain, you must do this.

4. Postponing tasks until the last minute

Since you enjoy completing tasks at the last minute, this bad behavior is much worse than procrastination. It causes an adrenaline spike, which is why. You could lose all you have, including your family and friends, if you continue this bad practice.

Even while it may make you feel enthusiastic to complete things at the last minute, it may annoy your loved ones. By making sure that you begin working on projects in advance through preplanning, you may overcome this bad habit the best manner possible.

5. Concentrating on the Bad

Individuals who have a tendency to focus primarily on the negative experience only bad things in their lives. Bad habits keep repeating themselves in this way. You become more immersed in this terrible habit the more you try to break it.

Counting your blessings rather than the bad things happening in your life is the best thing you can do to quit this harmful habit. By doing so, you may focus on the good things, which will eventually help you break the harmful habit of dwelling on the unpleasant.

6. Multitasking

Working on a report, browsing the internet, calling a customer, and texting your boss... excessive workload

Quit attempting to accomplish so many tasks simultaneously. If you attentively and sequentially do each task, you'll finish your work more quickly. Make a quick to-do list on a sticky note to get the activities off your mind if you're worried you'll forget what you need to complete. It's then time to start working.

7. Loafing

Real effort is one of the most difficult and evident aspects of accomplishment. Making excuses, procrastinating, or deceiving oneself into laziness will only serve to confirm that nothing will ever be done. The quickest path to success is to simply get started. It might not sound appealing or even too simple.

8. Blaming

"I'm not to blame for my lack of achievement. The market is poor, I lack the funds, etc. But who, in the end, is really to blame for their success? Themselves.

In today's world, people can build profitable start-ups in a matter of months, publish online, and find success in one way or another. Even while some circumstances may be beyond their control, blaming others would only squander the time and effort they need to start.

9. Unripe Grapes

Nearly as harmful as blaming others is being jealous of their achievement. You are devoting all the time and effort that you could be investing in achieving your own goals to someone who, more often than not, has done nothing more than convince you that your objective is feasible.

You don't have to celebrate their success, but it's a waste of time to be bitter and envious of it instead of working hard to achieve your own goals.

10. Minimizing the Success of Others

Again, you don't have to celebrate other people's success, but downplaying their achievements reflects poorly on you and your own objectives.

Would you want people to look at your accomplishment with contempt and act as if it weren't even a big deal? I seriously doubt it. Well, big whoop, they conquered Mount Everest. Many others have done it in the past. Has it been?

11. Making Preferences

You're aware of the proverbial saying that the word "assume" transforms "you" and "me" into an unsuitable term. The greatest at formulating assumptions without taking into account alternative options or opportunities are unsuccessful people. Anyone can fall behind or entirely ruin something they worked very hard on if they keep missing opportunities.

Individuals are frequently startled by what transpires when they take a chance rather than heeding that inner pessimist. Never assume is a wise maxim, and they ought to shed this frame of mind as soon as they can.

12. Investing Your Whole Day in Planning

Do you ponder how to make the most of each and every minute of your day as you study your schedule? Do you spend a lot of time making adjustments to Gantt charts and project spreadsheets?

Although planning is a crucial component of work, it is not the only component. You must also act and carry out the plans you have so carefully made! Set your plans aside and start working.

13. Sitting for Long Periods of Time at Your Desk

How recently have you taken a break from your desk? Unfortunately, using the restroom or obtaining a stack of copies from the copier don't count! You must take regular, unrelated-to-work breaks.

Give your eyes a break from laboring over your workstation or looking at the computer screen. Get up, stretch a little, then take a little stroll outside. Your body and mind will feel more energized thanks to the fresh air and scenic change.

14. Taking a Seat awaiting the ideal time to start anything

When would be the ideal time to begin organizing your closet, dream vacation, or job search? You might wait for the purported "ideal moment" for years on end.

The truth is that this very second is the ideal one. Quit holding out and get to work on your objectives, both big and small, professional and personal. You'll be happy that you did!

15. Reluctant to Acquire Fresh Knowledge

Learning a few new talents or approaches that are applicable to your line of work can be quite beneficial. These abilities don't have to be difficult; they can just be simple, commonplace tasks like learning to touch type, operate a copier, or resize photos on a computer.

16. Quitting

I tried, I guess. Yes, they made an attempt. As someone offers to climb back on it, the horse shakes its head and trots away.

Cutting losses occasionally is not necessarily a bad thing. No experience is ever completely squandered, but giving up is the worst adversary of the successful. There is no set path to success, only belief in what they desire to achieve.

You might need to clear your own route through a dangerous jungle. If they give up after the first mosquito bite, they are already doomed.

Success is largely influenced by the people competing. People applaud them for their hardship and success, but the person who scoffs while passively watching has never actually lived, either.

17. Negative Relationships

Some people desire a relationship in order to cling to that person. This is definitely not good. A poor relationship will occupy every square inch of your body if you do not want to end it.

This negative habit will try to stick with you even when you desire to break it. So, it is always preferable to recognize that you cannot change another person. The best course of action is to break up with a poor relationship as soon as possible.

You harm yourself and lessen your chances of meeting your soul mate by extending it. Discover why leaving a toxic relationship is a good idea and how to handle it if you're already in one.

18. spending time with cynics

You are frequently referred to as the sum of your organization. So, it is usually advised to form acquaintances with those that have a positive outlook on life. But, there comes a moment in life when you make friends with pessimistic people who have a tendency to turn down everything.

In the long term, this could truly wreck your life. The company you keep really defines who you are. So, it is usually advised to stay away from doubters because they taint your thinking and lead you astray. So, it is advised to become friends with those who have a positive outlook on life.

19. Too Much TV Viewing

When we were young, there were various outdoor games that we could play. But, as time goes on, we increasingly witness kids who are bored to death and glued to their television screens. They are now couch potatoes as a result of this.

Too much TV watching is a negative habit that can lead to laziness, obesity, and eventual predisposition to diseases like diabetes. The easiest way to break this terrible habit is to make sure you go for daily walks outside and set out a specific period each day to turn on the TV.

20. Angry Eating

Anyone in our day and age has stress, whether they are working or studying. Yet, when you use overeating as a coping mechanism for your stress, it develops into a destructive habit that must be broken. When we eat excessively under stress, it's often because we're preoccupied with the stress in our heads.

This causes us to consume mindlessly, which can lead to obesity and even diabetes. Never eating while watching television is the greatest way to break this terrible habit. Don't overthink your meals, too. Use your mind to process the food you are now eating.

21. Often Missing Meals

Water and food are both necessary for survival. Period. You probably aren't working as efficiently as you could if you don't consume meals frequently. Avoid skipping meals in favor of working and be sure you really enjoy your mealtimes. While you're at it, leave your desk or workspace and take a break from work by eating somewhere else, like a cafeteria, outside, or in a public park.

22. An unwholesome diet

A surplus of junk food (Including Diet Soda) Today, eating junk food has become a way of life. For instance, if both parents have started working, the children may frequently end up consuming diet soda and junk food, which can be harmful to their health.

With the current cultural shift, this is a really harmful habit that can be challenging to kick. The greatest solution to break this unhealthy habit is to make sure that everyone always eats home-cooked meals.

By doing this, the family's collective health can be protected. Nobody gets obese, which is a curse because obesity raises the risk of developing severe diseases like diabetes.

Well, but junk food is tasty, you might say. Toreconsider:

According to a study by Paul Johnson and Paul Kenny, consuming junk food affects brain activity in a manner comparable to that of addictive substances like cocaine and heroin.

Rats' pleasure centers grew desensitized to junk food after many weeks of unfettered access, leading them to crave more of it.

And you wonder why you seem to crave fast food when you just had some the day before?

23. A surplus of red meat

Red meat consumption is out of control, which is bad for our health. This unhealthy habit can cause us to consume too many difficult-to-digest proteins in our bodies. Our bodies were designed to consume a balanced diet.

Overindulging in red meat can ruin our appetite and make us susceptible to a number of harmful conditions. Red meat substitution with healthier protein sources is the greatest way to quit this harmful habit. By doing this, you can rest easy knowing that your health is current and that you won't expose yourself to any harmful diseases.

In addition, some studies have linked consumption of large quantities of red meat with breast cancer, stomach cancer, lymphoma, bladder cancer, lung cancer, and prostate cancer!

24. Biting nails

We have a history of developing negative habits dating back to our early years, and this is just another one. When someone yells at us or we can't get our way in adolescence, the added stress causes us to unconsciously chew our nails, which is a harmful habit.

The reason is that the nails that you bite get accumulated in your stomach, which can cause damage at later stages of your life. Biting your fingernails is a nasty habit that can be broken by dipping your finger in something bitter.

In addition to being unclean, nail biting is also socially awkward, causes dental issues such anterior teeth malocclusion, may result in stomach issues, and eventually results in horribly malformed fingernails.

In addition to having shorter nails than the normal person, those who bite their nails often develop scarring on their nail plates, which may eventually disappear.

Recognize the reasons behind your nail-biting behavior and switch it out with a neutral or constructive habit. Here's why you have to develop habits in order to break them.

25. Smoking

Smoking is one of the main global causes of death that may be prevented.

Our parents never let us get close to smokers when we were little. The reason is that smoking, even secondhand, is harmful to your health. When we become older and make friends with smokers, they tempt us to continue our harmful habit.

Your health may suffer, and it may even result in cancer. As a result, it is usually advised to avoid this dangerous habit of smoking. The greatest thing to do whenever you feel the urge to smoke is to put a pack of gum in your mouth.

This will help you break your terrible smoking habit. Male and female smokers, respectively, lose an average of 13.2 and 14.5 years of life; that's more than ten years of life right there.

Moreover, smoking results in early skin aging (wrinkles), tooth yellowing, bad breath, and, worst of all, endangers the health of those close to you, especially your loved ones. According to studies, non-smokers who are exposed to secondhand smoke run the risk of developing many of the same health issues as people who smoke cigarettes directly.

26. Extraordinary Drinking

People develop the harmful habit of binge drinking to cope with competition in the fast-paced world we live in. A few packs of hard beverages are not harmful to your health.

Yet, excessive alcohol use might harm your liver. Long-term drinking can lead to addiction, which is not beneficial for your lifestyle.

The National Institute on Alcohol Abuse and Alcoholism warns that excessive drinking, whether done once or often, can be dangerous to your health:

CONCLUSION

It's difficult to break bad habits. But if you make an effort to focus on the positive habits, these poor habits will fade away, and you'll escape the vicious cycle that is comprised of a list of bad behaviors.

Even though it can be challenging to change harmful habits, concentrating on positive habits will help you overcome them and improve your life in the long term.